Juicy Burger with the Works

How To Live Smarter:

A User's Guide

Rebecca M. Boys

Cover Contributors:

Grill Master - Neal J. Boys

Artistic Design - Brianna J. Boys

Photographer - Naleah J. Boys

DEDICATION

For my inspirational dad, Robert John Weinke, who during his most difficult fight still thought of his family, especially his beloved wife, my mom, Judith Ann and made sure his loved ones would be taken care of after he passed. There is nothing more important than family and the greatest gift we are given. Dad enjoyed preparing and eating delicious foods with his family, like a juicy burger with the works!

CONTENTS

ACKNOWLEDGMENTS

Set goals and take small steps toward achieving them. Things will not magically get done on their own. There is enough time if you make time for the things that need to get done. Writing is a hobby for me and I need to keep writing to get better at it. I think back to my dad's wish for me to create a cookbook of his favorite meals in remembrance of him with a gentle persistence. I know now he knew what he was doing to nudge me into something that I enjoy. It is important to have things that bring you joy and important for one's selfcare.

A few years after my dad's passing, my husband's parents gifted me with a writing course, which allowed me to earn six credits toward a Masters in Writing. At the time I was raising two young daughters, working outside the home, and never thought I could meet the demands of the course, yet I enjoyed the rigorous content of the material that made me write. I reflect back that I had loved ones directing me toward writing and I am thankful to have found my way back to it.

My husband's mother, Jan, is a writer who shared some encouraging words after my recent publication of *Why Not Live Smarter* that were worth mentioning as her unexpected review gave me insight to what others read. The "nuggets" or "jewels" as she called them are the foundation that these works are written on. It is how we choose to live and has worked well for us in raising our girls. The " jeweled nuggets" are as follows:

- Take time for yourself to rejuvenate. Slow down, rest and relax. Eat healthy meals together. Make time to be still. Listen. Enjoy the quiet times. Schedule in rest and relaxation having nothing planned. Read, write, and do puzzles being unplugged from the digital life.

- Be a team.

- Think blessed, not stressed.

- Love is what matters. Love is like wildflowers; it is often found in the most unlikely places-

- Faith, family and nature. Pray. Listen. Embrace aging. Promote wellness with balanced diet and exercise. Do not take yourself too seriously.

- Unplug and get outdoors. Breathe in the calm and tranquility of nature.

- Less is more. Commit and choose to be as debt-free as possible. Be content with what you have. Stuff weighs us down.

- Value education.

- Balance a full life with quiet, restful times. Seasons come and go; smile and enjoy the treasure in each one. This is not just seasons of the calendar year, but the seasons of life.

- Laughter. Be a bit crazy and laugh together.

Our world is too fast paced where she said the rest and relaxation in my book resonated deeply with her. It is not wrong, yet wise to reward yourself and family with play for working hard. It is hard for her to stop working when projects are not completed where she values that we do stop and play. I could not imagine raising our family and not having time together laughing. It is what made the journey worthwhile and created such grand moments in our time together. Our children grow in a blink of an eye and work will always be there; spending quality time together brings joy to all of our hearts, minds, and souls.

REV UP!

Create healthy habits, not restrictions. What initially was going to become a possible blog instead became a part of another eBook.

I live with hypothyroidism as a result from Grave's disease during my twenties. To save my life, I needed radioactive treatment to give me a slow metabolism. I ate well and exercised regularly, both of these lifestyle choices worked for me until my mid-forties. During the summer of 2017, at my yearly check-up, I received overweight papers and that was an abrupt wakeup call! I was sad and frustrated. I rarely treated myself to foods that I love, but are unhealthy (like ice-cream) and I felt that I did not eat too much. I exercised regularly and my clothes did not seem to fit tighter. I had gained fifteen pounds in two years and thought to myself what I would weigh if I ate whatever I wanted and chose not to exercise! Life is not fair and I am not a quitter so I saw this as another mountain to climb and literally that is what I did. With my family we hiked our first mountain that summer reaching the top at over 10,000 feet covering ten miles that day. If you understand mountain climbing that is a feat as we had done several half marathon

runs/walks/hikes on lower elevation and that seemed like a breeze to

climbing a mountain. On that hike, I began my thought process to

what I needed to do to stay in shape with my aging body that had a

metabolism of a crawling snail and the unfortunate genetic gifts from

my deceased father who passed away way too early. I wanted to try

and be around for my family and hopeful grandchildren. This may

seem a bit extreme to think like that, although it is not. I had spent

the last two years on a rigorous mammogram/ultrasound routine for

a suspicious area in my breast. I was on my last routine screening

that was moved from three months to six months before I would be

moved back to the regular yearly mammograms. This is when the

Radiologist requested a surgical biopsy as the area became too

unclear for his liking. Needless to say, as difficult as that was from

the procedure to waiting on the results, I had never been more

thankful to learn that my name had been moved from the urgent

mammogram reading list to the routine yearly screening list! During

the last two years I did a lot of pondering and praying while trying to

remove unnecessary stressors. Stress is the root of all destruction.

My father-in-law had told me that it was time for me to put myself first. My family was doing great and they needed me to care for myself like the way I care for them. He was right and it stuck with me. Listen to God's whispers and the ways they come to us.

I had successfully done a detox using the _Whole 30_ method. This helped me initially, however it is not a way to live, especially when I have my genetic gifts of naturally high cholesterol and triglycerides. I also read _Eating Right 4 Your Blood Type_, and that was the biggest eyeopener for me. Our blood plays such an important role as it travels to each and every cell, carrying the nutrients we need to feed our bodies. The blood type we each have affects the kinds of foods and drinks we should consume for optimal chance of health. Of course, I have the most difficult blood type of A+ that has very limited choices. Things that I would think to be good for anyone is not good for me. As an example, tomatoes have the wrong acidity where lemons are a better choice. I am learning gradually of what works and what does not. My doctor did not want a rash diet encouraging me to work on taking the last two years of weight off slowly for the best results. I did this for eight months, when I found out that I was only a few pounds lighter. I had a routine mini check-up for our health insurance that showed elevated blood pressure and that my blood counts were out of control. I always had great blood pressure except during my pregnancies which was due to toxemia. I learned during that time that one day it may return as a result. That day had arrived. My husband and I share the same blood type and genetic story. The nurse helping us that day said we're like siblings instead of spouses to how similar our insides are. Being blessed with facing whatever life throws us together; we would do just that with this one too. I feel my husband is better off in the weight department though as he has a naturally high metabolism. This is fortunate as he has hypothyroidism that we discovered due to him being tired all the time. A simple inexpensive blood test confirmed this which resulted in replacement therapy which helped significantly. Over many months his thyroid was regulated, which made him feel much better. One in four people have a thyroid dysfunction and it is often overlooked unfortunately. The thyroid controls so much within the body. I encourage any of you, especially women struggling with weight gain to follow along on my wellness journey as I share what I have learned. There are highs and lows in life requiring us to adjust to whatever we are given. My hope is that my story may help another to feel the best that they can, as life is hard enough. Go read these books and discover what foods your body likes the most so it can function at its best.

Rev Up! (but first pray…)

Goals work for me and being more determined than ever to bring my weight down, I set a goal. I not only envisioned losing the fifteen pounds that I had gradually gained, but I desired to reach my driver's license weight that was due for renewal. I made my goal specific to losing a total of twenty-five pounds. My current methods were not working so I began researching slow metabolisms in aging women due to hypothyroidism. I should have just listened to my husband as he said I needed to "Rev it up!" He said I did not eat a lot and I did not eat poorly yet I did not do enough to burn the calories I did consume due to my slow metabolism. He added that I did exercise regularly although not hard enough to get my metabolism going. I discovered that there was truth to what he said. I did discover though that I needed to add different food choices to help in the revving up of my metabolism. These picks would also cleanse my insides and try to rid it of anything that didn't need to be there. It sounds gross, but nonetheless it is true! I have always had slow moving bowels except during the Grave's Disease that was a huge indicator that something was wrong. I learned that my blood type basically should be a vegetarian diet. I enjoy meat and yes, a juicy burger with the works is a favorite for sure, except my recent blood counts showed that I needed to change my ways or a heart attack may be in my future. I decided to pick an assortment of fruits and vegetables then prep these for easy access. It actually was fun as together my family and I washed then cut the fresh veggies and fruit. My husband loves to cook so he began creating the best hummus using black and white beans instead of chickpeas as they are not a good choice for the A+ blood type. I eat salads for lunch using lettuce and spinach with a scrumptious carrot-ginger dressing (my husband also created this). We added hard-boiled egg whites removing the yolk to our salads then filled the egg whites with horseradish. Yes, here comes the part where you learn how to rev up your food! Use spices and a lot of them! I always cooked with your typical garlic, pepper and onion adding a few others depending on what I was making when I discovered that spices are the one thing that A+'s can splurge on. We had been grinding our own meat for quite some time already to help reduce the fat content, especially in ground chicken. It also is a lot cheaper to do it yourself. We now eat a lot more fish, especially salmon. It is more of a cost, however, that cost is minimal if you consider the medications you will need to lessen your sugars, cholesterol, and blood pressure if your diet does not work. Another switch to our eating habits has been drinking infused waters. The blends that I alternate in our home is a lemon, cucumber, and ginger with mint and a strawberry, cucumber, lime, and ginger with mint. We have always drank a lot of water so this was not a sacrifice and it quenches your thirst, while allowing you to easily drink a lot. I have always had warm lemon water upon awakening as it helps with sinus phlegm (sorry if this is too gross again, but this simple habit that makes me have less drainage as yet another trait A+'s are prone to have is more mucus) and my daughter encouraged me to add green tea and ginger to it. So, once again I revved up my diet by revving up my tea! Most recently we have begun brewing our own kombucha. We are not fans of the taste of the store bought kinds that are also costly. We understood the wellness benefits of kombucha, as it contains probiotics that help in gut health which helps combat stubborn belly fat. It is fun to grow our own SCOBY (Symbiotic Culture Of Bacteria and Yeast) and if you keep it in great conditions, it will keep multiplying from the original investment. Black and green tea are the best choices to brew with to promote high quality growing environments for the SCOBY.

The other habit that I stumbled upon was the use of Jillian Michaels' 7-Day Detox Drink. "Tea-tox" methods will help to hinder weight gain. It is important to stress that this is not a method underweight or even at ideal weight persons should do. You also need to be in overall good health with no life-threatening medical conditions. I will add that this is also for people who eat well, exercise, and get plenty of rest and still easily gain weight. It also is very important to keep up on the average person's daily water intake on top of the tea mixture. It is made from 100% unsweetened pure cranberry and lemon juice, water, and dandelion root tea. Simply brewed together for 10-15 minutes squeezing the tea bag to get the full benefit of the steep. I keep it refrigerated in a separate glass pitcher filling up a covered cup with ice and using a metal straw to sip on it continually throughout the day. You will be going to the bathroom A LOT!

Overnight oats have been in our routine for years. It took my husband some convincing to eat them cold in the morning as I prepare them the day before. I told him he could heat it up if needed when, low and behold he likes them cold from the fridge. My mother-in-law battles the same medical concerns and has a more rigorous meal plan than we do and suggested adding oat bran to our oat concoction. We did, thus revving up the "oaties"! I think you're getting the idea of where my possible blog name choice evolved from. I literally had to "Rev Up" everything in my life! It has paid off as only being down a few pounds in eight months and in the last two months I have dropped another eight pounds! I literally did a 180 just like that. I will say I am just starting to feel better as I was quite tired and sluggish as I only consume around 1390 calories a day as that is what is recommended from *MyFitnessPal* that my daughter also encouraged me to set-up and do. It really got me focused and it opened my eyes to what I am eating and getting my calories from. I am rarely hungry eating straight wholesome food. Grocery shopping is easy when the majority is coming from the produce section. I never ate much sugar due to being a borderline diabetic (another genetic gift or curse) so I am not dealing with sugar withdrawal as that is a hard process from what I have heard. A person truly does not need to eat a whole lot as drinking water is a key component to a body's health. I became hopeful that I could train my metabolism to work better. This is when I discovered that I may be able to help others that struggle with weight gain due to your genetic makeup that do eat well and exercise. (My oldest daughter and I have the hugest pet peeve with seeing others eat junk and nothing happens in the weight department although it will catch up with them.) I had shared earlier that my previous health issues made me remove unnecessary stressors so that I could add some things that I enjoy doing, like writing. It feels good to treat myself to something I enjoy. I just finished writing a family travel journal, as I had kept notes on our years of traveling the continental United States with our girls. That task had been weighing heavy on my shoulders for years and it was time to complete it. *Why Not Live Smarter Not Harder* was published in 2018. Create healthy habits, not restrictions and your life will become what you need. This results in the best version of yourself as you accomplish the goals you set! You also have to go easy on yourself if you are really putting in the effort as I never made my driver's license goal weight. I needed to add five pounds to my number from the last renewal which was ten years ago. My next license is due in eight years so hopefully I can take those five pounds off or it will at least be able to stay the same.

Breast Health & Wellness

Deodorant-no aluminum

Avoid plastic bottled water as it sits in the sun on loading docks

Use BPA free, glass or stainless steel water bottles

Use glass dishes for food at meals and storage

Do not wash plastic dishes in a dishwasher

Limit excessive heavy lifting…let others help

Use cast-iron skillets when cooking

Avoid too much sun exposure, shade yourself, be outdoors during

the better times of the day; and apply sunscreens as needed

Exercise daily

"You are what you eat!"

Daily Food Staples & Snacks

Back to the Basics; keep it simple!

Overnight Oats "Oaties"

Prepare an oat mixture (equal parts of ground flax, oats, and ground oat bran) be sure it is ground to be digested to its full potential once inside your body. We keep a big gallon size jar of the oat mixture ready to use. Scoop generous 1/3 cup of oat mixture into glass jar or bowl. Adjust to your serving size as needed.

Add chia seeds, nut choice-walnuts are our favorite and the best choice for our blood type (if you listen to your body it will prefer what is best for it), drizzle honey (local honey helps with seasonal allergies) and coconut water, skim or almond milk (non-soy) that has 4 times the calcium (people on thyroid replacement therapy should not ingest soy or mango as it will affect their medication from working properly).

Top with your frozen fruit choice (no added sugar), blueberries are our favorite.

There are endless options like adding peanut butter, but be sure it contains only peanuts and not all the additives, especially sugar. Cinnamon-Apple (use fresh) is a tasty concoction that we enjoy more during the fall months. For a special treat, frozen dark sweet cherries, cacao chips, and peanut butter are a scrumptious addition to the oat mixture, chia seeds, walnuts, and honey. Another spin to shake it up is adding frozen pineapple, unsweetened coconut, and cacao chips to the main mixture. Frozen, pure fruit with no sugar works best and is thawed by the morning.

Salads for lunch:

Guacamole, cottage cheese (Daisy brand is made of clean ingredients), pumpkin seeds, hummus, carrots, celery, peppers (all colors), banana peppers, dill pickles, beets, broccoli, peas (thawed frozen), dressing (vinegar or yogurt dressings as there are many healthier choices in stores), hardboiled eggs (just whites if you have cholesterol issues), and iceberg lettuce with spinach and kale (essentially any and all greens are excellent and tasty too with the right mindset, which is the key)

We eat oats & salads Monday thru Friday for breakfast and lunch. On the weekends we treat ourselves to egg whites made various ways, especially enjoying spinach scrambles from egg whites revved up with seasonings, as they are so tasty and filling too. Adding hummus, guacamole, and green salsa verde is a way to mix it up!

Snacks:

- Nuts/peanuts (watch serving size)
- Gluten free pretzels/whole grain crackers, so you don't get an allergy to gluten (portion control)
- Apple chips - homemade in the dehydrator due to the sugars added, although stores have some options but they are costly if it does not have additives
- Sweet potato & beetroot chips
- Lara bars

- Popcorn popped ourselves (pop and place in container or Ziploc as there is no salt and it is a lot cheaper)

- Splurge on any and all fruits & veggies

- Smoothies and juices are a tasty alternative with a good blender and the Ninja is highly recommended

Other Meal Staples:

- Veggie burgers with hummus and guacamole (be sure to avoid soy if you have thyroid issues and there are many non-soy brands in stores) topped with a fried egg is a real treat

- Fish tacos; simply prepare fish with taco seasonings and eat over a bed of lettuce occasionally serving with a small portion of corn or tortilla chips with salsa (green & red) with many of our salad toppings creating a filling and delicious meal

- Naleah's "Not Half Bad' Chili (recipe in the Rev Up Recipes section)

Everything in Moderation

Everything in moderation, including moderation…it's okay and necessary to treat yourself, even to splurge! You've earned it!

I do treat myself to ice cream as that is a favorite although I created a healthy "good for you" version to enjoy more often that is listed in the Rev Up Recipes section under Momma's Homemade Ice Cream.

Dig in the Dirt

Composting and gardening are two practices we have done for many years as a result of our oldest daughter's care and concern for the environment. We had that same mindset, yet it was her nudge we needed to make it happen. Out of the mouths of babes comes wise advice. Our world needs to pay more attention to their thoughts.

We have added a greenhouse to help us grow earlier and longer living in the Midwest with the harsh winter months. We collect and use rain water from barrels that we converted. Composting is quite easy where we use a small bin indoors then once it is full we just dump it into the garden during the winter. During the warmer months, we have a composter by the garden. We have the best soil from this practice along with rotating our vegetation. We have never had to use any pesticide and we are grateful for that.

Live Simply to Simply Live

Gardening has resulted in us canning and freezing to preserve our harvest so we can reap it throughout the next year. Recently, we were given an easy to make salsa that is canned. This recipe is found in the Rev Up Recipes section. Homesteading incorporating solar and wind power intrigues us. Protecting bees is something I am passionate about, as I know and am amazed at how local honey has helped the allergies in our family. Bees are crucial to the food chain. I absolutely love wildflowers so maybe in retirement I can do my part and add honey to our preserves in the process. It's fun to have goals and aspirations. Keeping life simple makes life full. To "Rev Up" your life is actually removing the extras that weigh us down from stress, calories, weight, negativity from others to our own thoughts, and anything that does not bring inner peace.

REV UP RECIPES

Cooking and baking healthier is a trial and error method. The following are some of our favorite go-to recipes that we find tasty and are fairly quick and easy to make.

Rev Up Recipe: Hummus

Hummus has become our protein staple. Many in-store brands are mostly made from chick peas and that is not the best option for A+ blood types. There are black and white bean options if you search harder although they tend to cost more. My husband is a natural in the kitchen and enjoys experimenting with food. Our favorite recipe for hummus is also the easiest to make.

Neal's White Bean Hummus

1 (16 oz) can white beans to 8 oz of garlic store bought hummus

Add ¼ tsp minced garlic

Blend together well (Ninja blender works great)

Store in covered container in the fridge

Rev Up Recipe: Carrot Ginger Dressing & Yum Yum

Combine the following ingredients in a Ninja blender:

3 washed and peeled carrots

½ cup water

5 tsp soy sauce

2 tsp rice wine vinegar

3 tsp sesame oil

1 inch of peeled ginger

Blend well and store covered in refrigerator up to one week.

Add 2 T. Thousand Island dressing (LITEHOUSE) to make it taste like a yum yum sauce that is a healthier version of it, and it's also yummy!

Rev Up Recipe: Brianna's Tater Tot Casserole

(Naleah's Campfire Creations or Daddy/a's Hobo Dinners too)

Brown 1 lb. lean ground meat choice with chopped onion, minced garlic, washed fresh mushrooms and pepper. Add a small can of non-fat, low-sodium cream of mushroom soup or low-fat cream cheese chopped into the meat using a little vegetable or chicken broth. Add drained cans of: cut green beans, corn, carrots and any other veggie choices to a greased 9x13 baking pan. Top with 1 bag potato or cauliflower tots. Bake for 45 minutes on 325 degrees. Top with shredded cheese choice if desired. (Cheddar and Mozzarella are both yummy) These are yummy placed in tinfoil and made over the open campfire too using small canned potatoes in lieu of tater tots, omitting the cream of mushroom soup for a healthier still tasty option also adding spices of your liking. Fish is excellent in the campfire option with fresh veggies and seasonings.

Rev Up Recipe: Momma's Easy Peasy Cookies

Mix together:

2 cups banana, almond or coconut flour

½ tsp baking soda

¼ tsp salt

2 tsp vanilla

4 tsp coconut oil softened

6 T. honey

Add cacao or any chips and or nuts of your choice if desired

Roll into balls

Place on greased cookie sheet

Bake 8-10 minutes at 350 degrees

To help harden the baked cookies; place in freezer for a few minutes.

Rev Up Recipe: Momma's Homemade Ice cream

Blend frozen bananas (we keep a container of banana chunks in the freezer to be ready to enjoy in that form or to be used in ice cream or smoothies) with a glug of almond or skim milk and another glug of coconut water. Add a generous tablespoon of natural peanut butter (no sugar) and a sprinkling of cacao chips. Adding frozen dark cherries and pineapple chunks is quite tasty too. Blend in Ninja and enjoy. So yummy. You can omit the peanut butter or cacao chips and just use bananas too. It also is tasty to just blend frozen pineapple alone with the milk and coconut water too. A satisfying and healthy treat is just frozen fruit unblended too. Adding whipped topping to any or all of this is always sweet and sure to bring smiles!

Rev Up Recipe: Papa's French Toast

Take bread of choice (the thicker the better)

Seasonal is fun to use too, like apple-cinnamon in the fall or dark chocolate chip in the winter or really anytime of the year!

In a small bowl, make a mixture of two cracked eggs, glugs of milk and orange juice, small drizzle of vanilla, and generous sprinkling of cinnamon or "simmer-on" as Papa would say.

Soak the bread in the mixture

Place on griddle or frypan until golden brown on both sides (flipping once)

Dusting with powder sugar

Serve warm with butter or peanut butter and pure maple syrup

My girls liked to add whipped cream and chocolate chips. Fresh sliced strawberries are yummy too!

Rev Up Recipe: Fabulous Fries

Wash and cut length-wise 3 big brown or yellow potatoes and/or sweet potatoes (can do circle slices using red potatoes too)

Place on greased baking sheet

Sprinkle with olive oil, rosemary, garlic and sea-salt

Bake on 375 degrees for 40-45 minutes

Rev Up Recipe: Canned Salsa (makes 6 quarts)

Doubling the recipe below will fit in a Nesco.

Combine in Nesco the following:

14 cups unpeeled chopped tomatoes

4 cups chopped onions

1/8 cup salt (optional)

½ cup sugar

4 cups finely chopped green peppers

2 ½ cup white vinegar

1 ½ T. chili powder

2 tsp each pepper & cumin

1 tsp alum

1/3 cup minced garlic

4 T. Tamazula

1 T. Frank's Red Hot

2 cans - 10 ¾ oz tomato paste

2 cans - 15 oz tomato sauce

Last 10 minutes add:

2 cans each drained corn & black beans

Cook on medium heat 1 ½ hours stirring often until thick. Put in

hot jars that were heated to boiling temperature. Add lids. Let cool

and check lids to be sure they all sealed.

Rev up Recipe: Grandma Jan's Kale Refrigerator Salad

Be sure to wash any fresh foods before combining into the mixture.

Combine:

1 peeled and chopped cucumber

1 cored and chopped apple of choice

½ cup shredded carrots

8 dried and chopped apricots (fresh peaches chopped up are tasty too)

¼ cup each unsweetened raisins, chopped walnuts or nut choice, and unsweetened coconut

Big bunch of chopped Kale

Mix together the following and pour over salad:

50/50 mixture of ¼ cup each of olive oil and balsamic vinegar **or** 100% beet, cherry or pomegranate juice (we prefer juice over vinegar, yet either are good)

Add a splash of lime juice

Toss salad together

Add cooked turkey or chicken if desired

Cover and refrigerate

Keeps for days or up to 1 week in the fridge

Rev Up Recipe: Nana's Banana Cookies

Combine 3 mashed bananas

1/3 cup unsweetened applesauce

2 cups oats

¼ cup unsweetened almond or skim milk

1 tsp each of vanilla and cinnamon

½ cup each unsweetened raisins, Ghirardelli 60% cacao bittersweet chocolate chips, and chopped walnuts or other nut choice

2 T. of natural peanut butter (just peanuts) if desired

Drop by spoonful onto greased cookie sheet

Yields 1 dozen clusters depending on size

Bake for 15-20 minutes at 350 degrees

So easy & tasty!

Rev Up Recipe: Pumpkin's Crockpot Chili

Grease crockpot and add:

1 lb. home-made ground chicken sausage no-salt or Jones brand is a better option to buy in the store (frozen from freezer works great just be sure to stir and break up before serving)

1 large can each pumpkin and green enchilada sauce

1 large jar white beans undrained

Chopped and washed celery, onion, mushrooms and cilantro to personal preference (two stalks of celery, big onion, large package of baby Bella mushrooms, and a big bunch of cilantro)

Pour huge glug of minced garlic from container

Heat on low for 8 hours or high for 4 hours

Serve with dollop of sour cream **or** plain yogurt and shredded mozzarella cheese

Rev Up Recipe: Salmon & Mashed Sweet Potatoes

Boil washed and peeled (if preferred) sweet potatoes then mash by hand or mix with hand mixer with a glug of almond milk, a sprinkle of cinnamon and top with pecans (if desired), which is delicious served with salmon. Place fresh salmon filet in pan on medium setting on the stove. Top with garlic and parsley adding any other spices of your choosing then cover and cook for about 15 minutes until inside is done to your preference. (Make sure it is done, but don't overcook as salmon is at its best when it is not overcooked and so tender!)

Rev Up Recipe: Fish Tacos & Cilantro Lime Rice

Place five frozen or thawed Pollock filets in pan atop the stove. Add glugs of lemon and/or lime juice and minced garlic, cover and cook until fish is done. Chop into pieces while cooking. Add taco seasoning and water if needed. Serve on bed of lettuce with veggies of your choice, such as: red, yellow, green, and orange peppers, onions, green and black olives, avocado, tomatoes, black beans, salsa, shredded cheese choice, and sour cream if desired. Serve with refried beans (there are many in-store low or no fat options) and/or Cilantro Lime Rice. Make two cups dry rice according to the package directions. Add washed and chopped cilantro and one tablespoon lime juice adjusting to your preference. Serve with tortilla chips. Easy and tasty meal.

Rev Up Recipe: Avocado Lime Rice

Make two cups dry rice according to package directions. Add washed and chopped cilantro and one tablespoon lime juice adjusting to your preference. Mix in one avocado. Add grated Asiago or Parmesan cheese. Enjoy!

Rev Up Recipe: Ella's One Pan Burritos & Taco Seasoning

 In the skillet heat: one can each of drained reduced sodium black beans, pinto beans and Ro Tel mild diced tomatoes & green chilies, cream cheese, and home-made taco seasoning or msg free packet. Heat and stir until cheese is melted. Serve in tortillas with tomatoes, avocado, onion, lettuce, cilantro, shredded mozzarella, and sour cream (Daisy brand is clean ingredients). Also yummy over Avocado Lime Rice recipe above or chips as in nachos.

Homemade (preservative free) Taco Seasoning

Combine and store in airtight container:

¼ tsp onion powder

¼ tsp crushed red pepper flakes

¼ tsp garlic powder

1 T. chili powder

¼ tsp oregano

½ tsp paprika

1 ½ tsp cumin

1 ½ tsp salt

1 tsp pepper

This has become a weekly staple being very tasty, easy, and quite healthy too. It is a win-win all the way around. Our niece, sweet Ella Bella, whom is also our Goddaughter shared this recipe. When she became married I had given her many easy and also good for you recipes with her surprising me with this treasure that she thought we'd enjoy also being good for Uncle Neal's dietary health.

Rev up Recipe: Sister Skillet Stir-fry

In cast-iron skillet, brown ground sausage of choice (Jones is great store-bought option) with water and a drizzle of olive oil

Add coleslaw or broccoli slaw in a bag (bought in produce section of store)

Season with paprika, turmeric, cumin, and curry powder

Crack 3 eggs into mixture

Heat a bit longer and enjoy with fresh avocado

Tastes like an egg roll except much healthier!

Our youngest daughter named the dish as big sister created this yummy delight that has turned into an easy standby for a quick and healthy meal.

Rev up Recipe: Naleah's 'Not Half Bad' Chili

(Naleah's comment when first trying momma's chili)

In a crock-pot, dump: 1 can each chili beans (undrained), corn, kidney and black beans (all drained), diced big can or fresh tomatoes, generous helping of minced garlic, 1 chopped onion, and chili powder to liking. Add glug of V-8 as needed. Cook on low. Corn meal or quinoa can be added and it is tasty. Serve with home-made Sweet Country Cornbread & adding honey is extra sweet.

Rev Up Recipe: Sweet Country Cornbread

Heat oven to 400 degrees

Grease bottom and sides of 8x8 glass or metal pan

Mix 1 cup unsweetened almond milk, ¼ cup unsweetened applesauce, and 1 egg

Stir in 1 ¼ cup yellow cornmeal and 1 cup flour (white or gluten-free choice-almond flour works well)

Add ½ cup honey (locally produced within 20 miles will help ward off seasonal allergies if faithfully consumed into your daily diet)

Combine 3 teaspoons baking powder and ½ teaspoon salt

Batter will be lumpy and be sure entire mixture is moist

Pour into pan

Bake for 20-25 minutes until golden brown and toothpick inserted in the middle of bread comes out clean

Serve warm and with a drizzle of honey…so yummy!

Rev Up Recipe: Sweet Potato Crust Pizza

Preheat oven to 400 degrees

Microwave 5 washed and fork poked sweet potatoes for 7 minutes

Potatoes will be very warm

(cool for a few minutes in the freezer if you want)

Peel potatoes and place in bowl

Add 1 cup almond flour

1 egg

½ tsp salt

1 tsp each oregano, basil, and garlic powder

1 T. apple cider vinegar

A pinch of chili powder

Mash with hands into dough

Use a rubber spatula to spread the dough onto a pizza stone

(be sure to spread evenly of about one-third inch in height)

Cook for 30 minutes

While crust is baking, prepare the toppings:

1 cup each rotisserie chicken and rinsed raw spinach

Sauté 1 thinly sliced red onion (uncooked works well too)

Add any other preferences:

Mushrooms, tomatoes, yellow, orange, or red peppers, banana peppers, and Italian seasoning

Remove crust from oven and cool for 20 minutes

Spread BBQ sauce of choice

(Sweet Baby Ray's any flavor is excellent)

Then top with ½ cup tomato sauce

Add toppings from list above

Drizzle with BBQ sauce and shredded mozzarella cheese

Bake for an additional 10-15 minutes

Slice & Enjoy!

Rev Up Recipe: Easter Traditions

We give up something of our choice usually any sweets, treats or junk

food like ice cream, chips, and fast food during Lent enjoying a little

splurge on Easter from goodies found on the Easter morning hunt.

It has always amazed me that our daughters from little on wanted to

give something up which is a testament to their inspiring beautiful

faith from little on.

Traditionally, we have hard boiled eggs from our creations dyed a day

earlier or boiled that morning with kielbasa sausage for breakfast and

a ham dinner for a "lupper" (a late lunch and an early supper).

Basically another Thanksgiving meal preparing ham instead of turkey

with many of the same side dishes as just once a year is not enough

to enjoy them, especially with the healthier variations created. I grew

up with the tradition of helping my mom bake and decorate an

Easter Bunny cake that is in my Dad's *Cooking Up A Cure For Cancer*

Cookbook (sold on our *Why Not Live Smarter* eBay account). We tend to decide what to have for dessert each year until recently I ran across a real ingredient from scratch Carrot Cake that we enjoy being a sweet splurge, especially since sweets have been given up for forty days.

Momma's Carrot Cake

2 cups shredded carrots (this can be doubled, even tripled for an extra moist cake)

1 (15 oz) can of crushed pineapple drained

4 eggs

¾ cups unsweetened applesauce

3 cups flour

2 tsp baking powder

1 tsp baking soda

2 tsp cinnamon

1 tsp salt

1 cup sugar (recipe calls for 2 although it is quite sweet with 1 cup; honey also can be substituted in place of the sugar)

1 tsp vanilla extract

1 ¼ cup olive oil

1 cup chopped walnuts

Divide batter into two or three circle cake pans depending on how many layers you would like or a Bundt pan is lovely too. Bake for approximately 45 minutes at 350 degrees or until toothpick tester in the middle comes out clean. More time is needed for the Bundt.

Cool and top each layer with homemade cream cheese frosting made from whipping 1 cup unsalted butter, 1 cup cream cheese, and 1-1 ½ cups powdered sugar. Sprinkle 1 cup crushed walnuts on top layer and or sides if desired. Simple, pretty, and yummy. Cake will keep three days covered in fridge.

Rev Up Recipe: Thanksgiving Dinner

Modified favorites:

Crockpot Mashed Potatoes:

Grease crock pot and add:

5 lbs. washed and cut red potatoes (peeled if desired)

½ cup each butter and Greek plain yogurt **or** non-fat sour cream

2 garlic cloves

1 cup each unsweetened almond **or** skim milk and low-sodium vegetable **or** chicken broth

Sprinkle with chives and ½ tsp salt

Cook on low for 4 hours

Serves 10 persons

Crockpot Green Bean Casserole (Brianna's favorite side)

3 cans of green beans

1 can non-fat, low-sodium cream of mushroom soup **or** low-fat cream cheese chopped into crock-pot

Wash and chop fresh baby Bella mushrooms (if desired)

Cook in greased crockpot on low for 4 hours

Roasted Cauliflower & Carrots

It is just that of fresh or frozen veggies placed in a glass baking dish then sprinkling no-salt spices of choice.

Green Giant **Riced Cauliflower Stuffing** bought in freezer section

Traditionally Basted Oven or **Nesco** or **Smoked Turkey**

Cranberries

Gravy (homemade from juices with cornstarch to thicken)

Nana's Pumpkin Pie & Whipped Cream (can from dairy section if time is an issue and also fun to decorate the pie or each piece with the can too)

Nana's Pumpkin Pie is from the recipe printed on most any large pumpkin puree cans. Prepare to recipe directions then pour into two deep dish pie crusts (homemade or frozen & baked first, both work)

Prepare **whipped topping** by combing: 1 c whipping cream, 3 T powder sugar, and 2 tsp vanilla mixing well with electric mixer.

Papa's Thanksgiving Prayer that we read and then share our blessings together around the table while enjoying a scrumptious feast and a "boomps" toasting one another with a clanking of glasses in glad cheer.

Papa's Thanksgiving Prayer:

We come to this table today, O Lord, humble and thankful and glad.

We thank Thee first for the great miracle of life, for the exaltation of being human, for the capacity to love.

We thank Thee for joys both great and simple:

For wonder, dreams and hope…

For the newness of each day…

For laughter and a merry heart…

For compassion waiting within to be kindled…

For the forbearance of friends and the smile of a stranger…

For the arching of the earth and trees and heavens and the fruit of all three…

For the wisdom of the old…

For the courage of the young…

For the promise of the child…

For the strength that comes when needed…

For this family united here today…

Of those to whom much is given, much is required.

May we and our children remember this.

Amen.

Rev Up Recipe: Christmas Traditions

Dig deep into your roots and share stories learning what has been in the family for generations

We found a dish from each of the nationalities we have: German, English, Italian, and Polish.

Rev Up Recipe: Nonna's Gnocchi Sauce

1 stick butter and 2 chopped onions sautéed until onions are slightly brown

Add large can of tomato sauce simmering for 30-60 minutes…the longer the better

Serve over gnocchi or any pasta with grating cheese if desired

Gnocchi can be found in grocer ethnic sections and we have begun to use, still tasting good using the homemade sauce.

Rev Up Recipe: Gramps' Tortelacci (pronounced "TUT–LOTCH")

In a large bowl combine and mix well:

8 oz cream cheese, 1 lb. Ricotta cheese, 1 cup grating cheese (Asiago or Parmesan) 1 egg, 1/3-3/4 cup bread crumbs, ¼-1 tsp nutmeg, ½ cup fresh parsley or 2 T. dry, salt and pepper to taste, 2-10 oz pkgs frozen chopped spinach, drained well

Chill. This much filling will take 5 eggs made into noodles.

Take ½ cup flour per 1 egg, plus a pinch of salt in large bowl, make a well in the middle and continue adding a total of 5 eggs to (making sure to add a ½ cup flour for each) working flour into the eggs by hand blending well

On floured surface, knead well adding more flour if dough is too soft to handle until dough is smooth

Carefully wrap dough in saran and seal securely so air can not get in for 1 hour before making noodles

Roll dough into 1/8 inch thick strips cutting dough into 2 inch squares filling with 1 T. prepared mixture until all filling and dough is used folding each square in half and pressing the edges tightly to seal looking like a Dutch hat

Place tortelacci in boiling salted water, cover and cook gently until dough is tender around 20 minutes

Drain and serve with **Nonna's Gnocchi Sauce** already written.

Rev Up Recipe: Babcia's Gołąbki (pronounced "GO-WUM-KI")

Remove the core from the head of cabbage (the bigger the cabbage the better) scald the cabbage in boiling water, removing a few leaves at a time as they wilt and cool before using

Stir ½ cup rice into pot of boiling water for 10 minutes and strain

Rinse with cold water in strainer being only half cooked

Sauté 1 finely chopped onion and 2 T. butter (don't overcook)

Combine 1 lb. ground beef and ½ cup pork sausage with 1 egg, rice, and any additional seasonings (garlic and pepper is tasty) mixing well

Spread the mixture into a cabbage leaf about a ½ inch thick

Fold the two opposite ends and roll, starting with one of the open ends fastening with a toothpick

Place cabbage rolls in baking dish and roast on 300 degrees for 2 hours then cover with **Nonna's Gnocchi Sauce** already listed.

Nonna's Gnocchi Sauce is a great choice to top off many dishes!

Truly a family favorite just like she was to us being such a sweet lady.

English heritage is remembered by all the sweet cookie treats.

German honored serving sauerkraut with sausages and brats. We

also boil up some spaetzle served with a drizzle of butter atop.

Polish is really done right with a batch of cheddar perogies served

with crushed cornflakes combined with melted butter to serve atop

the perogies. To enjoy the holidays by having more time to play games together too, we purchase and prepare *Mrs. T's* perogies.

Remember everything in moderation including moderation, we have modified the family favorites, but Christmas is the perfect time to celebrate the gift of Jesus with one festive party with excellent eats!

Countdown to Jesus' birthday with opening little gifts each day of Advent and our girls, both so appreciative of each gift they received stemmed from this special and sentimental tradition when they were quite young. Holiday Baking and the memories made through rolling the dough, cutting the cookie shapes and then decorating will always fill my heart with joy as both my girls enjoyed that special time together each Christmas season. You then create such a lovely platter of sweet treats to give to others and to enjoy together. Some sweet favorites of ours include:

Rev Up Recipe:

Minty Oreo Bark (one of the easiest and most delicious barks around)

Line baking sheet with parchment paper

Combine 25 oz white chocolate chips, 1 tsp coconut oil, and a few drops green food coloring (if desired)

Microwave on high for 25 seconds at a time; stirring between times until all chips are melted

Add ¾ of 20 crushed Oreos of choice (mint are yummy) and 1 tsp peppermint extract folding into mixture

Spread evenly across lined pan

Top with remaining crushed Oreos and drizzle with ½ cup semi-sweet cacao or chocolate chips

Place in the refrigerator for 2-3 hours then break into pieces

We also enjoy white chocolate dipped mint Oreos sprinkled with white decorating crystals and gluten-free pretzels drizzled with white chocolate. So simple, yet so yummy! Naleah's sweet delight for sure.

Rev Up Recipe:

Daddy/a's Chocolate-Covered Pea-nutty Pretzels

Line a large baking sheet with parchment paper.

Mix together 1 cup natural peanut butter and 2 T. unsalted butter softened to room temperature

Stir in ½ cup powdered sugar or bit more until dough thickens

Roll dough into 30 small balls adding more powdered sugar if too sticky then sandwich balls between two pretzels (square shaped pretzels work best)

Place on baking sheet and freeze for 20-30 minutes

Melt chocolate for about 1 minute in microwave, stirring every 20 seconds for the best results

Dip frozen pretzel bites halfway into chocolate and place back on baking sheet then refrigerate for at least 10 minutes to set the chocolate

Store in covered container for 10 days in the refrigerator or for 3 months in the freezer. Enjoy!

Rev Up Recipe:

Brianna's Moscow Mules (keeps well for weeks in the freezer)

In freezer-safe container add & stir together the following:

1 limeade or lemonade frozen concentrate

4 cans of your choice of: ginger beer, lemon-lime soda, ginger ale, or lemonade

*If you prefer the mixture to be alcoholic then add 2 cups vodka.

Scoop and serve alone or top with any of the above cans of choice.

So easy and a refreshing twist to any celebration!

CROSS-CONTAMINATED

It's not about you! Too many people make everything about themselves. The reality is that we are given the gift of life to give back, whatever a person's faith. For me it is that my God loves me just as equally as He loves anyone else. We are to use and share our talents we were graciously given and to not expect anything in return. Our Savior wants the best for each and every one of us and He has our back so we can have each other's backs. Kindness matters. Love is always the answer. Kind people are my kinda people.

Our world has become so self-centered and self-serving. Faith has become contaminated by these selfish ways. People in power say they are this religion or that religion and are behaving anything but humanely. Actions speak louder than words. The meaning of life is for it to be meaningful. Through giving of ourselves we will find happiness and fulfillment. By having less so others can have more is generosity at work. A person truly does not need stuff to be happy. Happiness comes from liking who you are and what you do. It is a personal choice. It is not another's responsibility to make you happy; it is our duty to live a life that makes us happy.

Everything happens for a reason. There is a lesson to be learned. Faith in that will carry a person through anything. God wants us to have a remarkable life! It may be difficult in the darkest times to see that, yet it is important to not lose faith. Try to keep watch for a glimmer of light to lead us on. Always have hope at your side.

Attitude
Charles Swindoll

The longer I live, the more I realize the impact of attitude on life. Attitude to me is more important than facts. It is more important than the past, than education, than money, than circumstances, than failures, than successes, than what other people think or say or do. It is more important than giftedness or skill. It will make or break a company, a home. The remarkable thing is, we have a choice every day regarding the attitude we will embrace for that day. I am convinced that life is ten percent what happens to me and ninety percent how I react to it.

Calm Chaos

- Life is chaotic if you let it be that way!

- Calm the chaos to what is best for you and your family.

- Simplify what you can, say no to keep your family the first priority.

- Use your crockpot or nowadays an instant-pot if you prefer to allow healthy eating as we are what we eat.

- Make cleaning your home a fun family activity by cranking up the tunes and going to town or doing little bits throughout the week makes it seem like less too.

- Losing your cool happens although harsh words cannot be taken back. Words matter, so speak wisely. Take time to breathe and think before you respond. Walk away if you need to. We try to not swear in our home and it has served us well. Try to know your limits and listen to those limits. We also try to not get to the point of yelling. This does not mean that we do not disagree. It means we communicate and sometimes agree to disagree. Our feelings and our family is what matters.

Joys of a Compassionate Heart

(ABC's of Life)

- **A**ccept responsibility

- **B**elieve in yourself, go beyond your comfort zones

- **C**reate lasting relationships

- **D**are to be brave

- **E**nter unfamiliar places for those truly in need

- **F**ind the right fit for your gifts

- **G**ive back

- **H**ave a heart of gratefulness

- **I**nspire compassion in others

- **J**oin the team of givers

- **K**indness is the key

- **L**ight a fire in others

- **M**agnify the magnificent

- **N**urture the ones truly in need

- **O**ptimistic outlook

- **P**ay it forward

- **Q**uiet your troubles

- **R**espect people

- **S**mile

- **T**riumph and learn from your failures

- **U**nshakeable faith

- **V**ictorious effort

- **W**isdom to do what is right

- **X**O XO (LOVE is the answer)

- **Y**ou can do it

- **Z**est for life!

BEFORE THE STORM

Dancing in the Rain

"Life is not about waiting for the storm to pass, it's about learning to dance in the rain." We follow this motto in our home and it helps us get through any of the unforeseen storms that do happen. Some of our most precious moments are when we literally danced in the rain with our girls, splashing in the mud puddles. Of course, we made sure there was no lightning!

It is easier than ever to capture the milestones of our lives. The digital age has phones in our fingertips literally and figuratively. Personally, I feel it is crippling us as a society if it is not monitored. Photos, videos, jotting notes through talking apps are a breeze and quickly captured. Scrapbooks revamped, email accounts to unborn children, letters from loved ones and a vast array of more clever and innovative ways to remember moments in time. All of which are ways to make life a bit more manageable. I wish I had some of these easier methods earlier in the raising of our girls although I'm at peace to what we were able to capture. (I guess I'm an old soul.)

The different stages of life and parenting if you decide to bear, foster, or adopt a family brings bountiful blessings among challenges. There is usually a calm before a storm and raising a family is no different. Trying to be prepared is awesome although most things just happen and you need to go with it. How you handle tough times is demonstrated through your actions. Remember that your kiddos are watching and listening.

Parenting Products

Focus on the needs (the essentials) not the wants at the different stages as it will help the family budget and instill the value of money from the start. The most beneficial product you can give your child is yourself. Your time and talents are needed to teach them from the start that they matter and that they are a priority to you. You show that through yourself helping them learn their worth and talents to then share back with the world.

Embrace the tiredness with your newborn infant as it goes by very quickly and truly is a critical bonding time to make the older, stress-filled years easier to know what your child is needing from you. It is truthful that little kids have little problems and big kids have big problems. There is much information available to what is truly needed and what can serve multiple uses growing with your child through toddler, preschooler, and even into school-age. The best gift you can give your child is to listen and then listen some more. Children go through much in today's society and parents need to be available to listen and to always love them. Tween and teen years are filled with much change physically and emotionally. Bigger the child is, the bigger the worry, the bigger the issues, and the bigger the parent needs to be there to help and guide their children into adulthood.

You need to help your young adult transition amidst many choices to what is the best route for them to be happy and successful in their life. Did you prepare them to handle the life skills (cooking, cleaning, laundry, finances, let downs, etc.)? Is immediate workforce or military entry, learning in an apprentice environment, attending a trade school or college-bound the best route?

College is not for everyone and if it is the path chosen, many hurdles lie ahead: Scholarships, Entrance Exams, Admission Letters & Deadlines that are both exciting and stressful. If accepted, many decisions lie ahead from what college to attend, how will it be paid, to the dorm room essentials and what is really needed for the space you are given. All of these things are new stresses requiring communication and plans of action to accomplish the steps involved to go the college-bound route. It is a big deal for your child to venture out on their own and also overwhelming so be sure you are there for your child. The world is amazing and quite scary at the same time. We wrote letters from us to our daughter to read while away at college and she appreciated them more than we even thought she would. It truly is the little things in life that show our loved ones just how special they are to us.

How quickly time passes; nursing my girls and transitioning them to our table food, from the clatter of pots and pans being arranged into skyscrapers with the help of food storage containers and boxes of all sizes (some of the best and least expensive toys) by your young artists and engineers, truly being some of the best moments in time. So simple and so rich in finding joy in the ordinary. Be present and be available to your child in the good and the bad so any storm that passes through will not destroy the family foundation created over the quality and quantity of time shared together. Family rooted deep in love and faith stays strong amidst the heavy winds of life.

Greek Proverb

A civilization flourishes when people plant trees under which they will never sit.

How glorious is the thought to enjoy caring for our family and to also think of others yet to come when we are long gone from this life!

PASSING ON

Traditions, stories, advice, experiences, lessons learned, and anything that a parent wished they would have known are all things to pass on. Life is not always rosy and should not be portrayed that it is. It is important though to not make adult responsibilities a child's worry. It is a parent's duty to be responsible to provide and care for their children. It is a parent's job to give their children roots and also wings to fly.

In establishing the roots creates the foundation of love and a safe haven for them to belong. Instilling the confidence to fly comes from teachings along the way. Simple life skills as in chores at age-appropriate times, easy recipes to make, the value of money, running a washing machine, apologizing for mistakes, accountability for inappropriate behaviors, manners, and all the little things that adults need to know to be successful are a parent's duty. Parenting is a huge undertaking and should not be seen as anything slight of that. Our kiddos deserve the best as it was not their choice to be here. It is a growing fact that more and more children, youth, and adults have mental health issues. Society and our values is the cause. Poor nutrition, lack of exercise, excessive screen time, friending instead of parenting, and an array of stuff all play a part. Anxiety is a result of the basics not being met. Our children deserve better.

Take time to slow down and connect with one another. Families are spread so thin and their schedules distancing. It is vital to make a living. It also is equally if not more important to keep your family connected. Is there a meal each day you can share? If not, there definitely is a meal to share at some point each week. There better be time made to check in on one another. That is where today's technology makes it quite easy, almost too easy that face to face communication is being lost. Once there is a time for all of you to share together then be sure to be present. Phones off. That simple.

Food is a comforting way to connect us to our loved ones. My girls still enjoy home-made French toast. It is a childhood meal my dad made for me and also taught me to make. It is something I passed on to my girls, now calling it, "Papa's French Toast." This recipe is found in the Rev Up Recipe section.

Do It Anyway
Kent M. Keith

People are often unreasonable and self-centered, forgive them anyway.

If you are kind, people may accuse you of ulterior motives, be kind anyway.

If you are honest, people may cheat you, be honest anyway.

If you find happiness, people may be jealous, be happy anyway.

The good you do today may be forgotten tomorrow, do good anyway.

Give the world your best and it may never be enough, give your best anyway.

For you see, in the end it is between you and God, it was never between you and them anyway.

Embrace the Gift of Time

The aging process is a journey of laughter and tears from both sadness and happiness. Embrace the gift of time shared to receive the effects of growing older. You have the choice to stay young at heart and that is truly your choice to make.

The best gift given to me was when my husband and oldest daughter were okay with me to let my hair be how it was, naturally almost white. I felt such peace as dyeing my hair was no fun, time-consuming, and not good for my hair or my health either. My youngest and myself were at peace with it. It was just hair and with what I was going through, I was thankful to have my hair. I have always saw white hair as pretty and I'm thankful to have healthy, long hair that I now can grow easily to donate and repeat as a way to give back.

Graciously Giving Back

We raised our girls to be generous in monetary and non-monetary ways. It is important for kiddos to learn from the start that kindness and helping are the best assets a person can share. In recent years after graduating from the Financial Peace University our daughter, Naleah, earns commission for her help in chores. We had chores from little on for both our girls although we did not do allowance faithfully as it was an expectation to help one another out that worked well to teach life skills and satisfaction from knowing every family member has worth. Since ourselves becoming more knowledgeable about finances, we see the worth to putting money regularly in their hands to manage. Our oldest, Brianna, is not quite sure she did not get jipped, in not ever having us do commission with her. Part of Naleah's commission is given away, another part saved, and the last part for herself to do as she wishes. No matter how small our contribution is, we try to help if we see a need. All on her own without us encouraging or suggesting, Naleah knew exactly where she wanted to help this Christmas. She did not just want to use what was to be given , but what she had for herself too.

Generosity at its fullest and the true meaning of giving to help someone in need.

The Boys Family Giving Project is something we have enjoyed doing through the generosity of my husband's parents. Money is given to each family to use to help a cause or a family in need. There is always a need and people should not look the other way to another's hardships. If every one did what they could, our world would be brighter.

A tradition for our first-born began at Christmastime for her to receive a little gift for each day of Advent. The cost was minimal as the purpose was to help her understand our faith with excitement for Jesus' birthday and the gift He was to us, the true meaning of Christmas. The joy she experienced each day to open her gift along with her sister then experiencing the same anticipation. So much more came from this little tradition. Both our daughters are appreciative for any gift they receive at any monetary value. I know it stems from this tradition we did with them. They looked forward to that special daily gift and what it meant. On Christmas morning they also received some gifts from Santa of course.

Thankfully Taken Back

Decorating for the holidays is a part of many families traditions. We were taken back by our insightful teen daughter asking us the following question:

"Why do we have to wait until after Thanksgiving to decorate when we're thankful for all we have?"

Why do we have to wait is correct! Such brilliance comes out of the mouths of babes. Traditions can be modified. We enjoyed preparing for the upcoming holidays with such ease and peace not feeling rushed.   We did little bits when we were able. The extra time was such a comfort. Listen to your kiddos and what they are sharing. Their thoughts matter and should be treated like they do.

When we are no longer on earth with our family, "What is it that you want your children to remember about you?" I certainly hope they remember all the love, laughter, silliness, and spur of the moment crazy times like seeing a commercial for a Culver's burger before bedtime realizing it was time for a run to the Culver's drive-through then enjoying the burgers together in their parent's bed.

And of course, those burgers were juicy with the works!

Another hope is that our children make the most of their dash as it is an incredible gift. In all the de-stuffing of having and keeping too much stuff the following piece was found. It is of much thought and treasure to share. (My husband wrote this in a reflection activity after receiving his Masters going on to take more classes to work his way up the pay grade.) Years prior, he was moved by a night show we saw in South Dakota that talked about the "Dash." What I found in his notebook was entitled, "3/5/73 - ?"

One dash, that is it. One little line. All accomplishments, experiences, hardships…everything, one day written with one tiny line. What will that represent? There are many different areas to look at. As a son and brother first, then as a friend, husband, father, then teacher, Uncle, co-worker, community member…a lot of stuff to fit in one line.

Am I on track? Have I started drawing that line in a way that I want it to look? Am I taking the time to enjoy the moment rather than be thinking about what is next? Am I making connections with the people along the way? Forgiving the wrongs? Treating people the way I should? Enjoying the time of the present? Spending the

time where I should, physically and mentally?

When the time comes to complete the dash and add the end

date, what is it that people will remember? What would I want them

to remember?

Parents: Caring, thoughtful, responsible, happy, kind, enjoyed

life, helped people, active, family orientated.

Brothers: Family orientated, active, good provider for family,

easy-going.

Wife: Caring, loving, romantic relationship driven, selfless,

funny, sincere, good provider, passionate family orientated.

Kids: Responsible, loving, family orientated, active participant,

concerned for well-being, well balanced with fun and discipline.

Co-Workers: Dependable, caring, dedicated, yet balanced

humor, good rapport with student also good control, organized.

Students: Connected, interested, fun, yet disciplined, model of

good living.

Are these the things they will remember? Will my dash look like I want it to? Are there areas of improvement? What can I do to get there?

Do not live the day to get through it. Live the day to live it. Enjoy it. Embrace it. Feel it. Hear it. Smell it. Taste it. Every moment. Every experience. Every encounter. Live it with no regrets. If you were done drawing the dash today, make sure people will remember you how you want them to. Don't bank on tomorrow, next week or next year to do it. Take care of it today. Stay focused in the present and the task at hand. Enjoy all the senses with each new adventure whether it is big or small, fun or not.

Take every moment that is in your dash and live them to the fullest and fill your dash with as many moments as you can. "Be patient toward all that is unsolved in your heart and try to love the questions themselves…Do not now seek the answers which cannot be given to you, because you would not be able to live them."

Do not live the day to get to the end, live the day to enjoy all the moments from beginning to end. There can be many questions and problems that use up all of your mind. Many of these questions and problems are without answers. The answers are simply in the way we live. They are in our daily mindset. They are how and who we are, not answers to put on paper.

It is far too easy to get caught in letting your mind torment about things that will not get you where you want to be. Past hurts. Re-thinking situations in the past over and over. Getting worked up time and time again about what you no longer have control over. It uses all of your mind's spaces and leaves your feet going nowhere.

Enjoy the Now

It is necessary to learn from the past, to let it guide you in the future. But it needs to be left in the past.

-Students-

It is far too easy to spend countless hours thinking of ways to torment that "student," that one that is "fingernails on the chalkboard." So much time can be spent in the past thinking about what they have done rather than using that and thinking about improvements that can be made.

Let it Go Make it Better* Be the Bigger Person*

If they punch you in the stomach, stand up, take a breath and ask them how you can help their day.

-People-

People can suck. Okay, I understand. Don't take it personal and move on. If your time is spent on what people have said or what they have done to you, you are not living for the moment. Your mind is in the past and you are missing the now. Now is when we are living. Now is when we are breathing. Now is when we are sensing the world around us. We will never get "now" back, so live it to the fullest.

FINANCIAL FREEDOM

Live within your means and you are on your way to financial freedom. Financial Peace University is an incredible program that set the path for us. It is something we have taught our girls so they will be in better shape from the start then we were.

Simple Smiles

Simple Smiles was a newsletter snail mail subscription sharing minimal or no cost family activities, traditions and easy & healthy recipes that I did as a way to earn a bit of extra income with two young daughters. It was blogging before blogging was a thing according to my girls' realization. I write of this to remember the ways we made ends meet connecting it to writing and sharing things that brought joy to our family without breaking the bank. It puts a smile on my face to all the simple times shared. It is extra sweet to remember my dear grandma being my first subscriber whom also encouraged me on my way to writing. I simply was sharing what I was working on during a visit with her. She was frugal with her hard earned money and insisted on buying a subscription for all her grandchildren that had families of their own. This was not expected and certainly a boost of confidence. I hope in retirement to compile all those monthly newsletters/calendars into something for free viewing to encourage families to play and laugh together without breaking the bank!

Simply Sweet

Christmas 2013 took us to our family in the South. Sitting around the dinner table, Grandma Jan brought out some toffee. Personally, toffee is not a favorite due to being sticky and hard to chew. This toffee was delicious and enjoyed by all! Gramps shared that the recipe was a secret and never shared by a friend of theirs who makes the toffee. We had hoped that at least her family knew the recipe, as it is a treasure unlike any toffee we have ever known.

 Our family helped at a local luminary event and we saw Sonnie who makes the toffee. I thanked her for sharing some of her toffee with us and told her that I have never really enjoyed toffee, but hers was different. We went about placing the luminaries and finishing up when Sonnie said to myself and my older, quiet child that she wanted to share her recipe with us. Gramps was shocked as Sonnie does not share her recipe.

My oldest daughter and I went to Sonnie's home for a lovely

afternoon with her. Sonnie wrote and explained her recipe to us. I

inquired if her family had her recipe and she said they did, which was

comforting to us. During our time with Sonnie, I shared that her

toffee would be a nice touch to my cookie trays at Christmastime

each year. Sonnie shared that "I do not want this shared with

anyone, because I want you to do what I wished I had done when I

was your age and turn this into a business". Upon our departure,

Sonnie stated that she felt my younger daughter would be a part of

this too. Sonnie knew nothing of our child's passion to find an on-

line business. I asked Sonnie if the recipe was a family tradition

and it was not. Sonnie touched my hand and looked into my older

daughter's eyes, then mine and shared:

I received this recipe much like I am sharing with you today about 40

years ago from an elderly friend. My friend made me promise that I

would not share her recipe until much time has passed and when it

felt right with the right person. We thanked Sonnie for wanting to

share with us and promised to not share her recipe until much time

has passed and when it felt right. I asked Sonnie what we should call her recipe as she had no name on the top of her written paper.

Sonnie was unsure and I wrote, "*Sonja's Sweet Toffee.*"

My older daughter and I took in the moments with Sonnie and

shared with family who all agreed that we needed to make the toffee

with Sonnie. Sonnie had thought the same thing and together the

three of us made toffee. Sonnie shared with us her inside scoop on

what makes great English toffee. Sonnie let us know that she

had wanted her recipe to be called, "*Sonja's English Toffee.*" I said that

at the right time I will call it that. Sonnie very kindly, but firmly

insisted that we do not let this opportunity go as she wanted us to try

and sell her toffee. Sonnie told us her research on toffee prices and

what she charges at her local bake sale each year.

During our long drive home, our oldest daughter formulated a

business plan to begin with and shared it with us. Both daughters

were determined to see this adventure through in honor of Sonnie.

Life is truly a journey that takes us on unexpected paths

and some are *simply sweet.* We did put in some effort researching and

realized that a commercial kitchen was needed. Brianna did

formulate a business plan with design and layout of the necessary paperwork that is ready if the future places the right time to pursue Sonnie's wish for us. The extra sweet note is that Brianna went on to earn her MBA in college showing signs of a business mind much earlier. Sonnie has passed on to be reunited with her husband although her sweet toffee lives on bringing smiles of delight.

Why Not Live Smarter eBay & Amazon Direct Publishing

Latest side hustles, including these eBooks. Minimal costs to sell and publish what you want. Biggest expense is your time involved.

Surviving Stress

Stress affects us. Stress is a part of life. No one is immune to it. The key is managing it. This process will be different for everyone simply because we are all unique. For me, I am a natural organizer which helps me greatly. I figure out what all needs to be accomplished and I create a list. This list contains my personal and professional responsibilities. Each day I get things done to the best of my ability. A few years back I had a huge wake-up call that I was not doing a good job managing my stress with learning that I may have breast cancer. Cancer thrives on stress along with my already less than desirable genetics which are prone to cancer. This showed me that I needed to put my own health first which is hard for me as I am the caretaker of everyone. I learned that I needed to give attention to myself and that was not selfish, but the right thing to do. My family needed me. I wanted to be physically around to see our girls' lives unfold and to enjoy our hopeful grandchildren. I realized that I needed more time to just relax as I tend to just keep going and doing. I needed more of something I enjoy just for me. My family is my everything although they are growing and needing me differently in their lives. In our home, we are a family that is a team. We decided that it was time for Momma to remove some of the stuff that could be dispersed better among all of us, or remove it completely, which eliminated any unnecessary stress.

I work outside the home in a high-stress profession. After much prayer along with myself being open and honest with my superiors, my work duties evolved to involve tasks that I mostly am able to do from home. God is great all the time. All the time God is great. I enjoy the work I do and I really did not want to find another less stressful job. I could help with the operations of the organization while not having the daily demands of the facility on my shoulders. I also am on the homestretch of retirement with over three decades working in the child, youth and family field. A graduate of UW-Madison in Family & Consumer Education with a business emphasis has placed me in occupations that first and foremost allowed me to be the main caregiver to our daughters. My husband and I believe that if the parents want to do the majority of the raising of their children then that is the priority. It was not easy as I found myself in high responsibility roles still caring for my girls while juggling those tasks. I am a positive person by nature so I believe my way of thinking helped me handle the dual duties of work and family for as long as I did. Good thoughts create healthy results. I tried to remain positive and to keep living through the unknown, but so grateful when I learned I did not have cancer. I think my body just got tired from helping everyone else and it was time for my own self to be my focus. That is not easy for me as I am a private person that truly enjoys helping others although I have realized with much reflection that it also can be quite exhausting. A doctor during my breast health routine shared that having too big of a heart in helping others all the time can be a harmful thing to a person's health. During this time, I pondered my stressors, both good and bad. Stress can be a very healthy thing in your life too if you enjoy the stressor. I was in a three-year term serving on a new board creating a children's museum. Although it included a lot of stress I enjoyed being a part of something that could have a huge benefit on children and families for a long time. I decided to finish my term, but not to continue into another term. It felt good so I knew I made the right decision. I had helped create a framework for the policies and procedures along with helping shape the education and exhibit committee which would allow the next member to build from where I had left off. Lastly, as a family and some unforeseeable experiences we resigned three months early from our church board serving on missions. It did not feel right to any of us and we believe in trusting your gut and that is what we did. Again, this decision to end our term did feel right and brought immediate peace to all of us so we knew it was the correct choice. God will place you where you need to be and as difficult as it may seem much joy is always just around the corner. He gives us free will and sometimes you have to just make a tough choice that feels right and have faith through the unknown process.

This is when we decided to hammer out our financial stress. We have always worked hard and with our chosen professions we would never have high earning salaries. We spent too much on credit in our early years of marriage, and our eyes were opened when we started planning for our future retirement. We always paid our bills, but we wanted better for ourselves and better for our girls so we educated ourselves and gained knowledge we wished we had known at an earlier age. We decided that we would teach our girls what we did not know at their ages. Anyone can be a millionaire if you decide you want to be one. It will take work, but you can do it no matter how much you earn. The key is living within your means and making your money work for you. My husband faithfully listens to talk radio, especially the podcasts of Dave Ramsey and Clark Howard. We have completed the Financial Peace University course and it is one that we highly recommend as we are accomplishing our own financial freedom. We also use the *EveryDollar* app that shows exactly where every dollar goes. We use a modified envelope system although we used it devotedly in the beginning that really helped us see the value of our hard-earned money. You think twice about paying with cash that is in your hands instead of simply swiping your debit card.   Our girls will be in better shape than us, but that is what you want for your children, right, to surpass yourself and have a greater life? In

reaching our goal to retire when my husband is first able to receive

his pension which is within this decade at fifty-five, we knew that a

side income would be helpful. This is also the same time our

youngest entrepreneur daughter shared that her online eBay business

(Why Not Live Smarter) was getting to be a bit much for her with her

rigorous virtual education she does. She added that I was the one

that helped her create and set it up and that it would make sense for

me to just continue with it. It did make sense and she is such an old

soul with such wisdom for her young age. First I destuffed our home

getting rid of any items of value to others. Then with much research,

along with trial and error, and with the limited amount of time

available currently, I learned that flipping jeans is worth my time and

effort. There is money to be made. It is crazy how much people will

spend on items and being the frugal person that I am there is nothing

sweeter than finding a great deal, except sharing it with someone in

need. My girls and I have become quite the brand new jeans finders

in stores. I take photos showing the details of the jeans, including the

tags that are attached and list them on our site. I put a fair price that

is much less than the cost to a person buying them in the store at full cost. I have the buyer pay for shipping. I use free mailing envelopes and boxes from the postal service. It really has become second nature and quite minimal in effort. I enjoy it also being something I would give more time to in retirement. Truly, think of your interests and skills using them to benefit yourself and family. I never thought my enjoyment of bargain shopping could make extra cash for my family and also help others in the process who enjoy shopping online.

I am still tickled pink that my simple bucket list project to journal our trips discovering the 48 states together and some other bits of moments in time into a keepsake for my girls has made us extra income. It is something that didn't seem to be of an interest to others as I was compiling it. The support from others purchasing *Why Not Live Smarter* did however encourage me to want to write something that may be of interest to others and possibly help them make the absolute best in their own personal life. I then felt I would be ready to finally tackle the beast of a piece that is decades in the work. My writing skills improved by putting out a few pieces and brushing up on my own unique style and voice.

LITTLE THINGS

Little things are the key to making life sweet and full of joy for our loved ones. Holidays and birthdays are no-brainer times to show our sweets their worth. It is at times of need the whole year through that little things matter. Is there a chore you could help your spouse with? Fold the laundry for no reason at all. Stop and pick up some groceries and start supper first. Motivate your family to do an outdoor hike in the woods together. Treat the family to a meal out or a movie together. Little things also become big deals. The big deal is building a sense of commitment and love toward our most special people.

Little things on a daily basis are truly the biggest things to a happy life. This practice shows your loved ones through action that they matter and you respect them to do things that bring them joy. This is just a little section, yet deserved to be a section all its own reaping some of the most special blessings in a person's life. I believe wholeheartedly that if everyone put care and concern on their own home front tending to their families, what a beautiful world we would live in. I leave this section with an abundance of ways to show your loved ones, especially your children just how special they are to you as actions speak so much louder than words.

Smile a lot

Acknowledge their presence

Giggle and laugh a lot together

Ask about their day (the good & the bad)

Look into your dear one's eyes when you talk with them

Listen to what they say even if it is not what you want to hear

Listen some more

Play a lot (indoors and outdoors)

Read aloud together

Embrace any feelings they share

Be kind and firm if need be

Set safe boundaries

Be honest and be yourself

Hug your loved ones for no reason at all

Forget life's responsibilities and worries to just enjoy your family

Listen to your gut and reach out if something seems off

Be helpful

Find solutions to problems together

Surprises are great

Surprises are extra special when you go on a hunt for them

Stay with them when they are afraid

Redirect inappropriate behaviors to promote better choices

Share excitement over their interests

Enjoy life

Write them a note or mail them a letter

Let them lead and you follow

Notice when they are not present, sharing that they were missed

Call or text for no reason at all

Give space and respect quiet time

Delight in their dreams

Be a comfort to any nightmare

Unwind and relax together

Be present in the moments

Try and answer or find answers to their questions or concerns

Look up to them, not down

Keep promises

Find joy in traditions

Hold their hand

Compliment genuine qualities

Apologize when you have done something wrong

Display their accomplishments, artwork, etc.

Use manners yourself

Let them have an opinion and respect it

Let them solve most of their problems with your guidance

Let them be little

Share your own struggles

Give them a nickname all their own

Be happy

Find joy

Praise them

Let them help you

Be flexible

Point out their uniqueness

Cherish milestones

Take a stand with them by standing at their side

Go on adventures

Do what they like to do

Be sincere

Let them have a voice in decisions

Dream big

Tackle tasks together

Help others that are less fortunate

Trust and believe them

Progress, not perfection

Go beyond comfort zones

Be an advocate of your family

Love them always, no matter what

A soul flourishes with good food, kind words, and laughter.

WHAT'S YOUR PURPOSE?

Why were you put on this earth? It is a gift and not something to take for granted. It is something to ponder if you have not. For me, I hope my purpose was to be the best Momma I could be to two remarkable human beings that I had the honor to raise. I also hope God has more for me as I'd love nothing more than to watch their lives unfold and to be here physically to help where I can. I also know my purpose is to help others as much as I can, even though I feel uncomfortable at times. I tried to minimize the chance of being put in very stressful situations, when I learned to embrace them as I can remain calm and find the positives in the situation. Keeping people safe is something I can and should do even if it is hard and difficult work. God will carry us through and I've learned to find reassurance in that. I continually meet struggling mommas and find myself uplifting and encouraging them, which is something that I have found joy in and realized that must be another of my purposes. From little on, all I ever wanted to be was a momma seeing it as the most important job in the world and that it is, definitely the most honorable privilege to care for the best gifts God gives us. I always wished I could have just been a stay-at-home momma and to not have to also work outside the home. Until recently, I have realized that God gave me the abilities to do both. I need to be thankful of my organizational and multi-tasking abilities. Our purpose is unique to each of us and we all have them. The key is realizing that we do and to embrace our gifts to then share and help when we are called to do so. Do whatever it is that makes your soul shine. If it is an occasional enjoyment of life's simple pleasures that is unique to you like savoring a juicy burger with the works, then splurge to your delight and do not feel guilty for doing it. You've earned it from constantly working hard and making healthy choices. Top it with all the fixings: cheddar cheese, dill pickles, raw and/or fried onions depending on the mood, fried egg, stoneground mustard, real mayonnaise, clean ingredient ketchup, and a pretzel or freshly baked homemade potato bun.

A favorite writing of mine is about a hundred years from now it will not matter what your bank account was, the kind of car you drove, the clothes you wore…But the world may be different simply because YOU were important in the life of a child. Encourage our children, others and ourselves. To love abundantly is a beautiful super power. Discipline constructively realizing and expecting that mistakes will be made by all that are involved. Teach your children right from wrong living by example as actions speak louder than words. Our children are looking and watching us all the time. Develop mutual respect. Listen. Really listen each and every day. Listening is key. Offer gentle, non-preachy guidance that fosters independence. The world is big and quite overwhelming so be the calm in the storm that is always there to lend a helping hand. To know that one person has breathed easier because you have lived is a success, and if everyone wholeheartedly did this then what a beautiful world there would be for our children and our children's children.

GET GOING!

Find your way to a better, more meaningful life. If there are obstacles in your way then start conquering them. Do whatever it takes to make you feel glad that you are alive. Life is a gift that most take for granted. Just waking up and seeing or being able to get out of bed on your own are things that many wish they could do. Become the best version of you for your own well-being and for your loved ones. You can do just about anything that you set your mind to. Exercise was my demise or obstacle depending on how you look at it. I enjoyed walking, but it was not working for me to maintain a weight I felt comfortable at. I needed to adjust my outlook and thankfully I had a motivating husband at my side.

Finding Joy in Exercise

Pick something you like or could like. It is best to have multiple choices to switch up so you can be better on your body. Yoga, circuit weight training, power-walking/light jogging, stair step/elliptical, twist board, ab ripper x, urban and nature hikes are all things that I use to reach my fitness goals.

My oldest daughter really wanted to do a half marathon with me which always was on the back of my mind too. Almost a decade ago already, my fortieth birthday was coming up. My very energetic, ambitious, iron-man finisher of an athlete, and sister-in-law, Kayla, was on it! She wanted to throw me a half marathon event to celebrate my 40th! It is quite cold in December in WI so she wanted to host it in TN where they had lived then. You got to have a sweet treat for your birthday, right; so it turned into a "Crazy Cupcake Run!" What a fun time it was and it gave me the motivation to stick to my exercise routine to not let my daughter or my sister-in-law down who had went above and beyond to make it a sweet time for all.

Our youngest daughter tagged along riding bike tandem behind Dadda helping Aunt Kayla, Uncle Daron and their young son, Gray on the course. Any help was always there by the capable hands of all of them working together to have an enjoyable time by all. Lovely, mini cupcakes were at all the water and fruit stops. The cool, damp and mists did not stop anyone as it was much warmer to us than most of the TN natives that still weathered the run.

Crossing the finish line with my sweet Anny (what I call my oldest daughter) was the best moment of all as we had done it together. I will carry that 40th birthday celebration with me as it was so unexpected, yet so delightful to have completed a difficult task with so much love and excitement for me to just do it. I felt so loved from the hand-made posters of loved ones there and also not in attendance. The natural wooden cupcake medals were simply delightful and a sweet remembrance. The fun long and short-sleeved designed t-shirts brought a real race day feel as well. The hand-made ceramic cupcake cookie jar made with love by Kayla and warm memories fill my being of all that moment in time held. She also made me one of her creative photo scrapbooks that is cherished. Brianna and I went on to do three more half marathons together until my knees and hips were hurting. It is important to listen to your body. I learned that I could run and actually began to enjoy it a bit. I am able to do short bouts of running, (which revs up my workout) along with power walking where that works for me currently. It was fun to do one of the half marathons in Madison with Daddy although he did the full marathon. It was so hot that the city opened the fire hydrants for the runners to have a way to keep cooling down. It also was an unforgettable time running another half with Daddy and Aunt Kayla sponsored through the Ice Age. Those inspirational running machines did a 50K as we accomplished another half that was certainly a feat for us being mainly in the woods and not always flat which we had become accustomed to. I had my sidekick and I felt I could do it and we did! Our half marathons turned into urban hikes of all-day power walking covering half marathon distances. We look forward to those hikes that now our youngest can do as well. It was a milestone moment when Brianna did her first half marathon without me. Her and collegemates ran in a Fall Hot Cider Hustle in Green Bay. As much as I enjoyed the time training and running with her, I held her back. I was proud of her to step out and accomplish it all on her own. Who knows what lies ahead on the horizon as our youngest wants to do something ambitious and is more interested in doing a "Tough-Mudder" together as a family. We have done several 5K races as a family so something a bit more challenging may be on the horizon. The key is to just get going physically, mentally, and spiritually to an abundant life worth living and to enjoy living it!

To "Get Going" is not just in the physical sense, but in the living life large sense too. There will always be reasons to not get going from financial, attitude, or exhaustion so make the choice to just go! It is the spur of the moment times that are some of the best moments in time. Recently, on our youngest's search for her college, it was learned that she will most likely need to attend college out of state due to her interest in becoming an Aerospace Engineer. Time is a ticking. We knew we wanted to take her to the places that interest her to have her experience firsthand the atmosphere of the different campuses. She had a different spring break than Dadda, but the same as cousin Hannah.   Hannah and her mom, due to unforeseen issues, had a planned trip they no longer could do so it was decided to take a mini road trip to begin tackling Naleah's college list. It is these all-girl road trips that simply delight us. It was just a few days although much laughter, miles, and memories were made together.

Leave A Trail

Do not go where the path may lead, go instead where there is no path and leave a trail. -Ralph Waldo Emerson

"Crack it around!" This is just an example of one silly remark that was said when the going gets tough and has become another lighthearted way in our family to deal with life and the difficulties we all face. Keep the humor and get it done one way or another. Crack it around and get going!

BUILD MOMENTUM

An impactful message we had heard was discussing new year resolutions and how most people fail at doing them. The talk went on to share the idea of having a vision. The vision included stackable moments that build momentum to achieve happiness one year from the present. It simply used the following question: What is the **one** thing I can do **today** to **build momentum** to bring **happiness** one year from now? You then applied that question to the following areas in your life: Spiritually, Physical Health, Personal Growth, Career, Relationships, and Financial. These small stackable moments are achievable and help you stay the course to your own personal happiness instead of becoming discouraged by unattainable resolutions made with no vision. We took the idea and created our own vision for our family in 2019. We were never a fan of resolutions, yet this idea intrigued us and it helped us create a vision that was attainable for our family. We used a laminated flyer-style copy of the info listed below that we could use dry erase markers for any revisions or thoughts we had.

2019 VISION BUILD MOMENTUM

What is the one thing I can do today to bring happiness one year from now in the following areas:

Spiritually - daily devotion & 13 influential Bible verses in a year

Physical Health - eat well & exercise faithfully

Personal Growth - no tv until after 7 pm

Career - BAM & CYA (our family joke to find the humor staying grateful for income)

Relationships - family first, using our strengths to help others

Financial - follow FPU with monthly budget

Under each area of our life we discussed things to bring happiness in one year from now as with most anything of worth takes time to see and feel the results from hard work.

Spiritually - daily devotion & 13 influential Bible verses in a year

We failed at personal and family devotion simply by setting unrealistic goals that we could not attain. As an example, we tried to read the Bible in a year falling short and being frustrated amidst our other life responsibilities. We managed to read parts of the Bible not enjoying it and finding that it is imperfect. Written by enlightened humans makes it imperfect to a revelation our youngest shared with us. We stopped our goal to read the Bible in entirety to finding time for a better relationship with God and our faith. We prayed our own way and that is enough. God wants to help us and not burden us to unrealistic resolutions, especially if you live a full life with minimal free time. Parts of the Bible are inspiring with impactful verses. Again, our youngest thought to find thirteen verses in the next year that we find meaningful and become familiar with them. We picked thirteen for prosperity into the next new year. We also like the number thirteen as a family. Fun Fact: My diamond engagement ring also has a total of thirteen diamonds. We were crazy from the start and certainly not superstitious as we have been blessed beyond measure for sure.

Verse 1: Song of Solomon 2:10   He calls me beautiful one.

This was a verse I had found on a cute wooden decoration block while shopping for Christmas with my oldest daughter. It was on clearance that was a bonus yet so simple and of truth. My girls are so beautiful from the inside out that it was the perfect find with just two left on the shelf. It is a great reminder to each of them to love who they are aside from what society says. They are both rare treasures with wholesome values that no matter what, they are beautiful always in our eyes and God's. It was also a reminder for myself that I'm beautiful in God's eyes too. How we see ourselves impacts our children. I always build them up with their gentle reminder to be sure I am building myself up as well. Again, how wise our children are. Much can be learned from their sweet voices.

Verse 2: Psalm 86:15 Thank you for being slow to anger.

This verse resonated with my husband on our daily devotion app. He is a veteran teacher with retirement on the horizon. It was not until a few years ago, especially the last several that he looks forward to retiring. Teaching is not just teaching anymore and understandably it frustrates him. Society has created a larger group of entitled young people which makes the career more difficult. There are the gems in the crowd; sadly those who want to still learn and to be challenged to their full potential are lowering in numbers. He feels more like a social worker than a science teacher. He is such an awesome teacher reaching many of the "hard to reach" kids although it has taken a toll. This verse reminds him how patient God is with him and in turn he tries to be that with his students even when they make it difficult from their lack of interest and disrespect. Sadly, the apple does not fall far from the tree and parents need an adjustment with an increasing number of students not having parents because of something on the crazy list of reasons. This only makes the obstacles even greater for young people to reach graduation and to be able to prosper in adult life.

Verse 3: Psalm 116:7 Relax & Rest

Our world is too fast-paced and there is a huge benefit in slowing down to enjoy the moment in time. We all deserve to relax as a reward for working hard. Compassionate people who care for others as a way of life often put other's needs ahead of their own. Do not allow tension to build up by having stress management and relaxation techniques as a part of your own wellness plan. There are quick ways to minimize stress like deep breathing. Close your eyes and breathe deep. Hold your breath for a few seconds then exhale slowly. Do this for as long as you are able, thinking about relaxing your body, mind and soul. Laughing out loud is an instant release of stress. Think of a funny moment in time, a joke that makes you laugh, or simply plan to watch a show that makes you laugh. Think about a peaceful place by closing your eyes and visualizing the place, smell the aromas, and hear the sounds. A few moments to stop and visualize a relaxing place can take you to a calm spot uplifting you for the tasks still at hand. Talking to a trusted source is a way to vent out frustrations and hopefully puts things back into perspective. There are many relaxing activities that are unique to all of us. It is always good when there is minimal cost involved to not create financial stress by thinking you are treating yourself when in reality it creates more stress. Some inexpensive ways to bring rest and relaxation into your life are as follows:

Light some candles

Aroma diffuser with pure oils & water

Go for a walk

Journal

Read

Sip some tea or hot chocolate

Take a country drive

Listen to some tunes

A bubble bath

Treat yourself to a meal out

Sing

Dance

Catch up with a true friend

Yoga

Enjoy a favorite hobby

Cloud watch

Stargaze

Meditate

Enjoy a movie (staying in or going out)

Verse 4: 1 John 4:4 The Spirit in you is far stronger than anything in this world. Stop "Stinking Thinking" and pray first taking the right steps forward to have your best year ever! Another great message we heard in church this past year.

Verse 5: James 1:19-20 So, then, my beloved brothers, let every man be swift to hear, slow to speak, and slow to anger; for the anger of man doesn't produce the righteousness of God. Oh, what a beautiful world if others slowed and practiced respect and kindness as a choice to make life brighter for someone other than themselves. This time in history requires more patience and care for one another. It is easy to become angry at life and how nuts it seems, yet we need to stay true to what we are, children of a loving God whom is slow to anger in all our faults. Find the good in others and build them up by helping them through their journey.

Verse 6: pray first - 21 days of prayer & fasting is a devotional of prayers that we did together at meal time to kick-off the new year. Praying is something we try to do first on the ups and downs in our life so this was a comfortable practice for us to do. Praying helps carry our worries and joys to the Lord which minimizes anxiety and stress knowing that He is with us and wants us to talk to Him. Fasting is something we do slightly during Lent, usually giving up sweets. Fasting at the start of the year was a way to detox after the holidays. Truly a person does not need a lot of food. Fasting is a personal choice and should be done with concern and under a doctor's care to be sure dietary guidelines are met. The key for us is to eat smaller portions of wholesome, healthy foods for your nutrients and to stay plenty hydrated by drinking water. These are two practices we need to do to stay as healthy as is possible year round. Giving up the extras is not hard as we already do not eat much junk food, however it is amazing to what a person does eat if you are more in tuned to it. A few gluten free pretzels here and a handful of peanuts there were discovered and minimized. We are enjoying the creative ways our worship is being shaken around a bit instead of the same routine practices. God is alive in us and we should want to share His lively spirit generously that is within all of us. God's timing is always perfect and we need to remember and trust in that.

Verse 7: Psalm 112 Message to share His light in the darkness knowing His presence is always with you to carry you through.

The word of the year for our church family is: Establish - to make strong. Our pastor's prayer for our church family: My prayer is that your heart is strong enough for the climb. The climb is different for all of us, yet God's love is enough to carry us through.

Verse 8: James 1:17 Every good and perfect gift is from above, coming down from the Father. How true this is and the most beloved is the gift of children. This verse arrived in the mail from Nana to Naleah on a lovely Valentine's card also etched with, "God gives us good gifts to remind us of His love for us." This sweet tradition Nana has done with all her grandchildren on both Halloween and Valentine's Day to remind them just how special they are. Nana shared that she decided to end this tradition with Naleah being her youngest and let her great grandchildren begin traditions with their grandparents. There is a season to everything. Naleah cherished the card realizing that Nana has had thought behind these cards and just how special she is to Nana. Nana has a special way of making all her grandchildren feel loved. Naleah is Nana's Pumpkin being born on Halloween. In the card Nana wrote, "You're one of the really good gifts and you're loved so much! Thanking Him for You. Happy Heart Day, Pumpkin. Stay like you are, SWEET. Love

You!" Naleah is extra sweet and unique with her way of making all feel loved and valued and she portrayed these qualities from a young age having such an old soul vibe. Our name choice was perfect for her as Naleah means 'A gift from God,' and that she is. As children are one of the best blessings, so is family, in whatever way it is given to us. Be grateful for the people God places in your life and the capacity to love and to be loved.

Verse 9: Romans 1:16 For I am not ashamed of the Good News of Christ, for it is the power of God for salvation for everyone who believes; for the Jew first, and also for the Greek. This daily devotional spoke volumes to my husband as we shared a bit of a Monday morning together before beginning another full week ahead. Spring was upon us finally after an extra cold winter. Either driving conditions or feeling under the weather kept us for several Sundays from church. We missed church and the uplifting energy it gives us. The daily devotionals on the app during the weeks we missed were nothing to write home about. The morning devotional after going to church resonated deep within him as he told me about it. I knew it definitely had to be documented as part of our finds. The pastor's message talked about speed bumps getting in our way of doing our best practices in life such as little lies turning into big lies and how we can justify doing wrong things. The speed bumps try to slow us down and are God's way to help us realize the wrong paths although we have free will. God will not strong arm us to do what is right as we have to want to do what is right. If you go too fast over the speed bumps you could crash or at least cause harm. The daily devotional went on to talk about a father in the park with his children along with other families gathered. The park was in coyote country so this dad in particular kept a close eye to ensure safety on his family. Most families present were not attentive and coyotes were spotted in the distance. The soft-spoken, caring father roared in a loud voice very out of character for him alerting the others about what he saw in the distance. His children were horrified at the spectacle their dad was making and no one listened as he roared again. This is like our Father who loves His children. He will do anything for us to keep us from harm's way. He also wants us to do everything to share His love for us, especially when others are not listening! He does not want us to be embarrassed of His love for us. It is a lovely treasure to share.

Verse 10: 1 Corinthians 16:13-14 Watch! Stand firm in the faith! Be courageous! Be strong! Let all that you do be done in love.

Our daily devotional talked about being utterly lovely in all you do. It also referenced Mother Theresa's thoughts on anyone can do small things with great love. Imagine a world where everyone was doing small acts to brighten another's day and being attentive to others in need. If you ponder a bit, life is really a bunch of small things put together to create our lives. If love is put into the little things of our daily life, what an utterly lovely world! The simple act of being patient as you are waiting, not becoming enraged when a car cuts in front of you, or the genuine use of manners. Love is in the little things. Love is a verb. It's action. It is the mark of being a true Christian. Our marriage ceremony was based on 1 Corinthians 13; sweet to see how impactful and utterly lovely more chapters are.

Verse 11: Hosea 6:3 "Let us acknowledge the LORD. Let us press on to know the LORD. As surely as the sun rises, the LORD will appear. He will come to us like rain, like the spring rain that waters the earth." Rain is so refreshing and life-giving to the blooming of spring. Spring break road trips have been a part of our family traditions many a time, usually with our favorites (Uncle Jason, Aunt Heather, & Hannah) and usually to some place warmer than our homes in the North. For many reasons the annual Spring Break trip all together did not happen and was missed by all of us. I thought about our missed trip as I read my daily devotional. We lose out on so much if we do not make time for God and the nourishing only He can bring. Be thankful for the beautiful people He places in our life and the times given to enjoy together. Needless to say that everyone already figured out their Spring Break times and another adventure together is in the works. Make time for the ones that bring life to your life. It is true as you do not know what you have until it is gone or missed. Family and true friendship is a most treasured gift.

Verse 12: Palm Sunday message was said and heard in a way we had never before experienced. Palm Sunday and the story shared many a time, yet never as impactful and meaningful. We absolutely love and enjoy our new church, feeling God in ways we never imagined. God wants us to live and experience Him in glorious ways! Our pastor spoke in great length about the lambs during Passover in the very early times of history. These pristine lambs became a part of the family for many days before being given to the high courts and only accepted if the high priest believed that the family truly loved and bonded with the lamb. If not, then the lamb was ordered to stay with the family until genuine care and love was shown toward the lamb. Our pastor brought a live lamb out for part of his message that was quite impactful with the creature bah-ing at opportune moments too. His message brought home the whole "PASS-OVER" of the homes with blood from the lamb on the doors. It just also shared the correlation of Jesus being our real Lamb of God. The Passover practice began much earlier in time than the birth of Jesus Christ. Jesus was the pristine lamb who came to allow death to PASS-OVER us. Jesus rode in on a donkey through the same gate that the lambs arrived in each Passover. Another twist in our family conversation after church that Naleah shared was about Peter, the leader of God's disciples. Just as the priest asked each head of the household if they loved their lamb for up to three times before a decision made, Jesus did this of Peter. Jesus asked Peter if he loved Him three times. God knew Jesus would die on earth for our sins and Peter would be leading His disciples. God wants us to love Him in a relationship with Him and not as a religion, but out of genuine love for Him with a good heart.

Dadda's take away was that Jesus spoke to Peter before Easter just like Peter is the name of the Easter Bunny! Faith is linked to the Easter bunny too. So God wants us, just like Peter, to hop His message of love to all the kiddos, big and small, on Easter and all through the year.

Verse 13: Philippians 4:8 Finally, brothers (& sisters), whatever things are true, whatever things are honorable, whatever things are just, whatever things are pure, whatever things are lovely, whatever things are of good report: if there is any virtue and if there is any praise, think about these things. Our thoughts are powerful and also have the ability to restructure our brain. God created us in hopes of thinking positive throughout life. This is not an easy task with all the hardship and yuck in our world making it hard to see and find the positive. Science shows through neuroplasticity that the brain has the ability to change and adapt throughout our lives. Every thought produces a chemical change in the brain affecting the overall structure of the brain. Negative thoughts may increase mental illness while positive thoughts improve brain health helping people to perform at their optimal potential. God wants us to live abundantly and positive thinking is key. Try to see the good in life and in others. Freely and joyfully build one another up. This devotion resonated deeply and truly felt like the best was saved for the last of our thirteen Bible verses. God never said that life was going to be easy, in fact just the opposite. The beauty is that He wired us in a way to cope and handle challenges. We are given blessings to be with us, Him among us, others at our side, and our choices to make the absolute best of our lives and time on earth. Life is hard for all, with mental illness at a high. A simple solution is thinking positively. Medication is not always the answer and may even be a negative path to wander down. Medication is needed in some cases, although it is not needed for just feeling down in the dumps. Sadness is a feeling all of us experience at times. We have the choice to think well, do well, and be well. We raised our daughters to live positively, even among hardship finding the silver lining that they witnessed firsthand by watching us through our actions. Life is certainly not easy, but it certainly is a gift meant to live victoriously!

Physical Health - eat well & exercise faithfully (One daughter had a personal goal to run a mile in eight minutes while three of us wanted to plank each day to lead to overall weight loss in one year.)

Rest & Relax was written here as a reminder to offset the hustle and bustle of daily life in the outside world. Our home is a haven that brings peace to our mind, bodies and soul to be able to tackle life in a positive way.

Personal Growth - no TV until after 7 pm (I personally delete emails too quickly, so to make my husband happy, it was decided that I move the emails to a folder then sort together into the trash each month when we discuss the next month's budget.) It truly is the little things! Instead of turning on the TV, we have free time to catch up on anything of our choice, be it reading, daily devotion, praying, writing, a puzzle, housekeeping, and etc.

Career - BAM & CYA (our family joke to find the humor staying grateful for income) Our daughters and us all work extremely hard, too hard. We attempted to keep things on the light side by finding the humor to make work fun and appreciating having the ability to work to have income and to get us where we want to be in the future. This also keeps life real. People can be exhausting with my girls and I all being introverts with my husband being an ambivert makes us all appreciate the quiet and calm of our home together.

Relationships - family first, using our strengths to help others (This is our family way and we honestly believe that if everyone put their families first our world would be happier and better off in so many ways.)

Financial - follow FPU with monthly budget and continue to grow our side hustles to help us retire at the earliest time possible.

We made and used a laminated copy throughout the year for easy reference. My husband also had a laminated copy of the one listed below on his bathroom mirror for easy daily reference:

What is the **<u>one</u>** thing I can do **<u>today</u>** to **<u>build momentum</u>** to bring
<u>happiness</u>
one year from now?

Spiritually - Physical Health - Personal Growth - Career -
Relationships - Financial

- Stack Moments –

May you find too that your vision of personal or family happiness is achievable with **stackable moments** of effort while building momentum to live smarter. Everyone has off days and that is what is so awesome about stacking moments that if you lack on any given day you still have your momentum to carry you through. The key is to strive for some success each day, no matter how small, stacking the moments keeping the momentum alive. Each day is a precious gift to be lived with a heart of gratefulness to the treasure it is!

ABOUT THE AUTHOR

Rebecca lives in Wisconsin where she cares for her family with the help of her husband, Neal. Together on their journey to financial freedom and faithfully tackling the challenges in daily life , they have learned to live smarter, not harder. She has written a *Cooking Up A Cure* cookbook in honor of her late father, Robert, poetry that has been awarded honors and published, and *Why Not Live Smarter, Not Harder* which was a bucket list project that motivated her to continue on in a hobby that she finds enjoyment in doing. After this piece, *Still Living Smarter, Not Harder* and a fantasy fiction are all in the works. In the meantime she continues *to work smarter so she can play harder* in retirement and remembers to indulge in life's simple pleasures savoring every bite of her occasional ***Juicy Burger with the Works***!